The Songs of Love

The Songs of Love

Dipraj

9 August 2020, 4:04pm

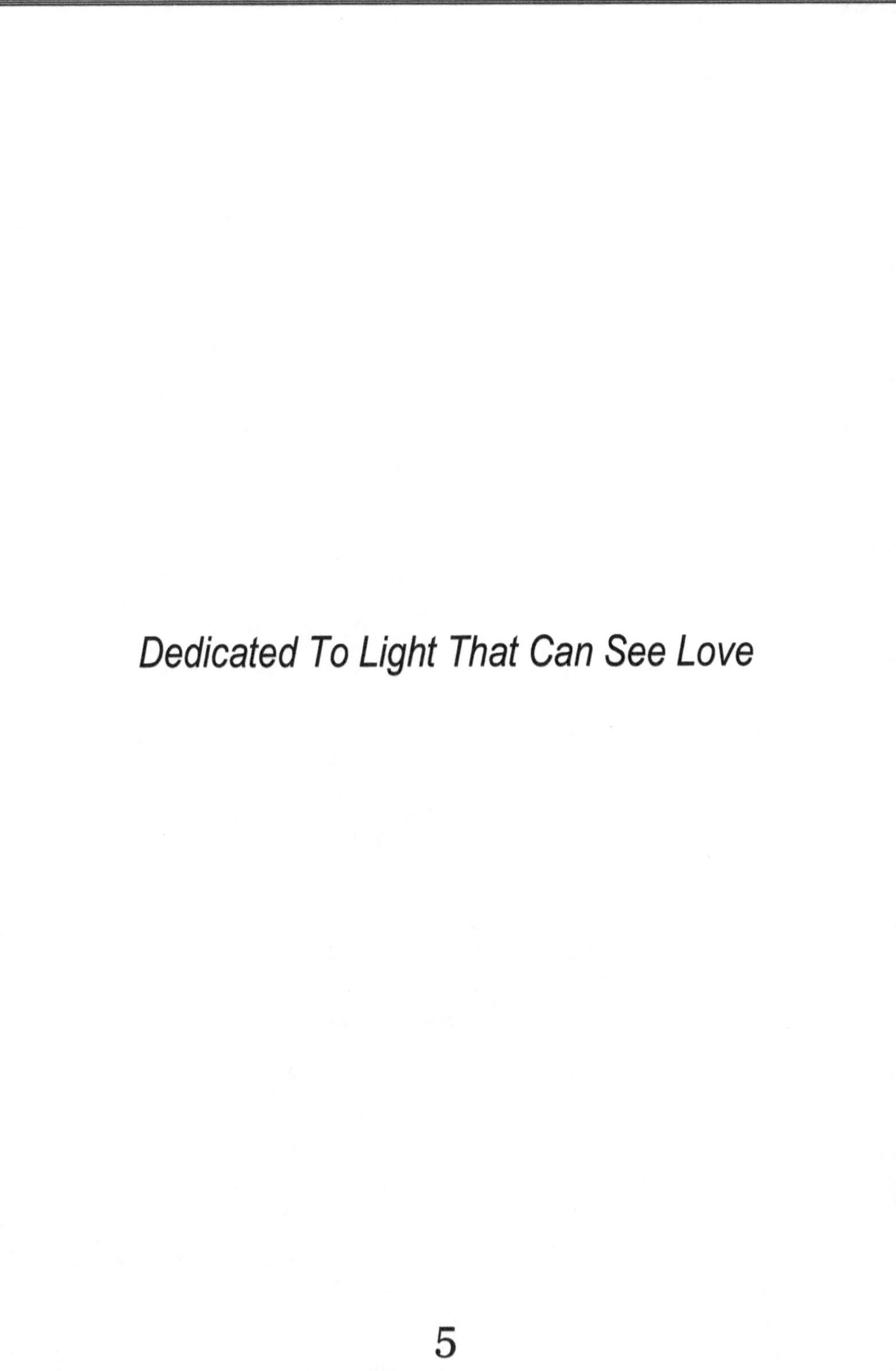

Dedicated To Light That Can See Love

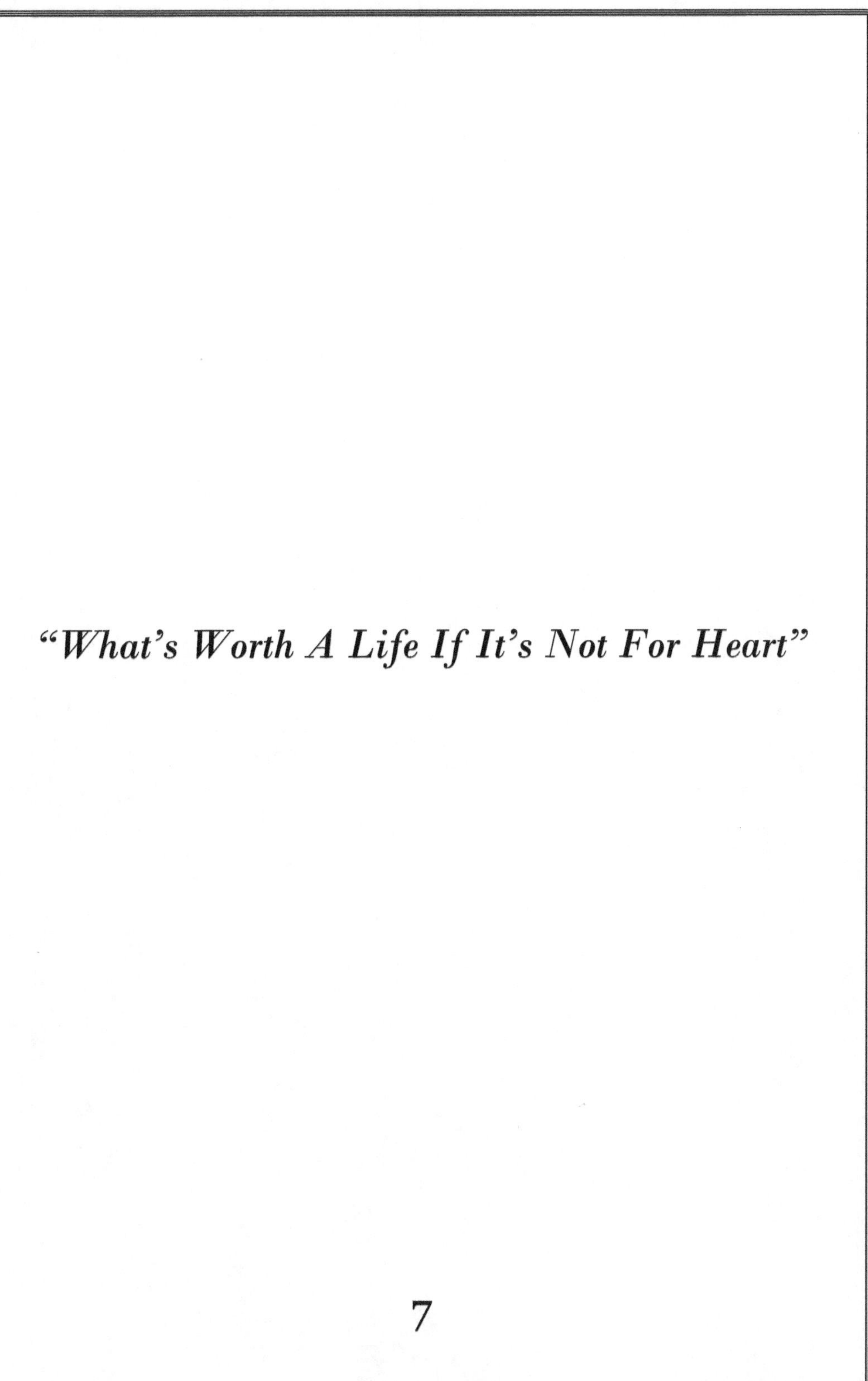
"What's Worth A Life If It's Not For Heart"

Table of Contents

Introduction

Love Does Not Need Introduction. Yet, You Who Have Lost Yourself Need To Be Introduced To Who You Are.

You Are The Light That Can See Love. And It Is Only Love You Need Ever See. It Is Only Your Choice To See Something Else That Has Made You Blind.

Love Will Never Abandon You. Neither In Time Nor In Timelessness.
Yet, You Shall Be In Darkness Until You See The Light You Are

Nothing Shines Without Knowledge.
The Spirit You Are Cannot Shine Without Knowledge - Complete And Whole.

Indeed It Is A Journey. But Why It Need Be Tough? Let's Sing The Songs Of Love In Your Heart. And Light Is Not Far Away!

I Wrote These Songs To Remind You Of Love That Is Everywhere.
Your Minds May Not Understand As Yet. But Your Hearts Are Ready. That's Sufficient!

Elements

"How Shall You Have Life If You Reject
That Which Makes Life?

Creator

There is The Ocean of Love
That Is Full Of Love
You Are But A Droplet in That Ocean
This is Creation

Who Can Really Measure The Ocean
And Who Shall Know The Ocean
For Only Ocean Knows The Ocean
And The Ocean Knows Every Droplet In It

You Are In The Ocean
That is Why Only Ocean Surrounds You
You Who Think Are Separate From The Ocean
But Only Delude Yourself

Be One With The Ocean
And All of The Ocean Is Yours
In Your Utter Submission
Is All Your Gain

Your Strength Is In Being Who You Are
And You Are Love
For Love Created You
To Extend Love

The Creator Of Love
Wanted To Extend Love
So He Created Spirits
The Light That Can Extend Love

He Also Created The Teacher
To Bestow Knowledge To Spirits
Thus, Love Light And Knowledge
Are The Eternal Ones

This Is Not The Only World There Is
For On the Surface of The Ocean
There Are Infinite Bubbles
And Your World Is One Such Bubble

How Do I Know All This?
For I Am A Destroyer of Bubbles
And I am going To Destroy This Bubble
To Return All The Droplets
To Deep of The Ocean

You Who Are Spirit
Believe The Bubble And Question The Ocean
Yet, This Is Only Ignorance
And Ignorance is an illusion

Only Love Light and Knowledge Exist
And All This Will Be Restored
To Your Awareness
And You Will Know Who You Are

You Are The Perfect Creation
Of The Perfect Creator
There Is No Death To You
For You Breathe Life Into Life

Yet You Do Not See Any of These
This World Seems To Be Ruled By Time,
Sickness, Death, and Ignorance
You Shall Overcome All These

You Do Not Really Live
Until You Understand What Life Is
You Do Not Really Be
Until You Know The Being You Are

I Cannot Tell You Much About The Creator
You Will Have To Meet Him Yourself
He Reaches To You Always
You Need To Reach To Him

He Isn't Far really
Closer Than The Breath You Breathe
In The Space That Moves Your Each Thought
In The Love That Rests In Your Heart

You Do Not Really See
Neither Do You Listen
But You Will See What He Shows To You
And You Will Hear His Words

Then You Will Realize
The Beauty That's There
That Which Is Yours
And What You Are Here For

Spirit Indeed You Are
Soul You Have To Fulfil
Heart You Must Treasure
Mind You Need To Free
And Body You Should Make Use Of

O Travelers of Love
Let's Complete This First
For In The Completion of This Journey
Is The Healing You Deserve

None Of This Is Hard
To Be Natural Is The Easiest of Things
You But Need To Decide
What You Truly Want

Yours Indeed Is The Journey
Back To Your Creator
For Only In Meeting Him
Will You Meet Who You Are

No One Can Avoid This Journey
You Think You Can Delay It
Think Again
For You Are Meeting The End Of Time

Love To Creator of Love
Love To The Light You Are
Love To The Knowledge That Shines
O Beloved! Love You Always!

Spirit

That Which Is Beyond Life And Death
That Is Spirit
Spirit Alone Can Make Life Alive
Spirit Is Deathless

Body Is Too Dense To Show You This Light
And Spirit Is Beyond Mind, Heart, Intellect, Soul And
Consciousness

Then How Would You Meet The Spirit You Are?
Only Your Creator Can Answer

Yet, Let Me Show You Some Signs
To You Who Are Too Attached To Your Body
Of that Which Is Not of Your Making
And That Which You Are Bound To Meet

Spirit Is Light
Unlike Anything You Will Ever Imagine
You Can See This Light With Your Body's Eyes
If The Creator Grants You The Grace

Spirit Is All Powerful
The Creator Grants Him Everything
Shred All Your Imagined Weakness
For It Does Not Exist

Spirit Is Forever United With God
The Created Never Separates From The Creator
The Illusion of Separation You Have
Is The Choice You Have Made In Your Ignorance

Spirit Gets All It Wants
The Creator Loves Spirit Beyond Measure
Spirit Is The Will Of God
That Will You Have

Spirit Is Ever Free
What Can Limit The Limitless
What Can Contain The Infinite
Who Can Dare Touch The Fearless

Fear Not What You Are
And Do Not Disgrace Yourself
By Calling Yourself a Human
You Are Not Human
I Am Not Human
We Are Not Humans
We Are Spirits

Body Shall Never Tell You Who You Are
And You Are Not Meant To Suffer In Body
All Your Pursuits Are Centered On Body
Center Everything for Spirit
And Everything Shall Be Yours

Does All This Sound Unbelievable?
Indeed It Is
For What I Tell You
Is Beyond The Domain Of Belief

Darkness Seems To Obscure Light
Death Seems To Rule Life
Give Up All This Seeming
For Spirit Is Perfect Certainty

You Cannot Know Spirit Without Knowledge
And You Cannot Have Knowledge Without Love
Love Is In Your Heart
Give It All And It Will Give You All

There Is No End To Spirit
But You Must Begin!

Mind

Where Do Thoughts Move
And What Do You Use To Create
What Can Bind You To Illusions
And What Can Free You To Reality
Mind Is The Answer

You Do Not Really Know Your Mind
You Believe It Is In Your Body
You Cannot Control It
And It Is The Master Of Your Life
What A Cost For Carelessness!

You Do Have A Mind
That Perceives This World
That Looks Outward and Sees Objects
That Which Causes All Sickness In Your Body

This Is But Your Lower Mind
The Storehouse of Suffering
The Place For Your Belief In Separation
The Kingdom Where Your Ego Rules

You Have Another Kingdom
Which Is Not Your Creation
This Is Your Higher Mind
And You Can Access It

Your Lower Mind Is What You Chose To Abide In
And Look What It Has Cost You
All The Perception of a Material World, All Helplessness, All
Doubt, All Loneliness, All Diseases, All Attack, All Concern
for Survival, All Fear, All Attachments, All The Belief In the
Power of Body, All Hate, All Indulgence, All Avoidance, All
Forgetfulness, All Misery, All Enmity, All Judgment, All
Confusion, All Distractions, All Avoidance, All Guilt, All
Shame, All Blame, All Meaninglessness, A False Sense of
Identity That Begins With The Painful Birth of Body and
Ends with Its Death Into Nothingness
This Is All You Ask When You Choose Your Lower Mind
As You Ask You Are Given

You Do Not Doubt This
For Each One Of You Experiences These Effects
And All of You Have Chosen To Suffer Together
That's Why You Share All These Effects
And This Sharing Makes All These Effects Real To Your
World

What You Refuse To Admit
Is The Power of Your Mind
You Are Too Careless About The Thoughts You Choose To
Keep In Your Mind
There Is Nothing Constant In Your Mind
That's Why The Beauty You See Does Not Last

You Do Have A Higher Mind
This Is The Mind Your Creator Shares With You
All Purity Lies In It
There is The Peace Of Immortality In It

You Can Undo All The Effects of Your Lower Mind
They Are But Illusions and You Can Dispel Them

But You Do Need To Learn To Train This Amazing Tool
An Untrained Mind Is A Disaster
A Well-Trained Mind Is Unparalleled Asset

How Shall You Train This Mind?

Start With Detachment
Learn to Detach Yourself from Everything You See, Touch,
Smell, Taste, Hear, Think, Feel, Believe, And Seem To Know

Detachment is Not Hard To Develop
All You Need Is But A Decision To Detach
And You Need Not Detach Physically
It Is Mind Where Detachment Is Needed

Then Comes Reflection
Reflection is The Ability To Mirror Your Thoughts In Your
Mind
And Play With Them Before They Go Out
Reflection Will Allow You To See Your Thoughts

Now Follows Contemplation
Once You See Thoughts
You can Meditate Upon Them
Investigate Them for What They Are
Contemplation Allows You To Go Deep Into Your Mind

Now Develop Awareness
Be Aware of What You See, Hear, Touch, Smell, Taste,
Think, Feel, Experience, Say, Do Not Say, Reveal, Hide,
Perceive, Believe, Complain, Communicate, Share, Withhold,
Give, Receive, Engage, Disengage, Indulge, Consume,
Expect, Give and Receive
Awareness Is Your Friend
Keep Him With You Always

You Are Ready for Mindfulness Now
Mindfulness is To Be With Your Mind
You Are Too Distracted By What Your Mind Shows You

Be Grounded, Stay With Your Body, Mind, Heart, Intellect,
And Soul
Mindfulness Has Wonderful Benefits
It's A Healing Medicine
Your Restless Mind Will Surely Appreciate
Teach Yourself How To Be Mindful

There is Power Of Appreciation
That Can Restore Mind To Beauty
Teach Your Mind To Appreciate Beauty, Grace, Kindness,
The Good and The Divine
What You Appreciate Will Find A Place In Your Mind And
Abide There
To Appreciate Is To Breathe
You Need To Do It Often If Not Always

There Are Limitless Powers of Mind
For Mind Is Limitless
The Ones I Mentioned Are A Good Start
Master These and Your Mind Will Thank You

Condemn Not Your Mind'
It Deserves Only Love
All The Ugliness It Seems To Contain
Are But The Effects of Your Own Choices
And You Can Always Choose Better

What Is Greater Than Greatest of Thoughts
And What Is Smaller Than Mediocre Thinking
Your Thoughts Are Seeds
Do Not Be Surprised At The Yield

Powerful Indeed The Mind Is
But You Are Spirit Whose Powers Are Above All
That Is Why Your Mind Is Completely Yours To Command
O Spirit of Light, Let Your Light Shine In Your Mind
Your Mind Needs To Shine
For You Have Hidden Darkness There
And That Darkness Is The Cause of Your Suffering
Prepare Your Minds For Light
And Light Shall Abolish All Darkness!

Heart

When Earth Was Created
Life Was Delighted To Find A Home For Her
But What Did Earth Want?
She Wanted To Love

How Would She Love?
For Even Though Most Tolerant Of All
She Was The Most Delicate
And There Was No One Who Could Understand Her Longing
For Love

So The Magnificent Creator
Created The Most Beautiful Thing
On Earth
That Thing Is Heart
You All Have It

O Beautiful Ones,
There Is Nothing As Beautiful As Your Heart
And In The Beauty of Your Heart
Earth Finds Love

And Like Earth You Too Long For Love
In Your Hearts
And There Is So Much Love In You
None of You Can Ever Contain It

O Beloved Ones
You Have But Misunderstood Yourself
You Think Love Is Limited To Body
That Only A Few Can Be Loved And Not Everyone
That Love Can Hurt
That You Can Love Only Sometimes And Not All The Time
That Love Depends On Language
That Love Can Be Rejected
That Love Can Be Restrained
That Love Can Be Judged
That Love Is Not Spiritual
That Love Is Bondage
That Love Makes Demands
That Love Is Attachment
That Love Is Yours To Keep
That Love Can Cause Pain
And The Worst of All
That Love Is Your Weakness

Such Is Not Love

And Your Heart Cannot Understand It
That Is Why In All Your Wanderings For Love
The Heart Of Yours Has Only Met Thirst

You Have A Gift In Your Heart
The Gift To Give Love
Each Time You Give This Gift
It Is Returned In Abundance

For Love Only Multiplies
And Grows With Each Giving
And In The Receiving of It
Is Your Soul Nourished

Yet Why Do You Not Experience This Truth?
For You Have Limited Yourself and Your Heart
And In Those Limits You Have Suffocated Your Soul

Do You Really Think There Is
Impurity In Your Heart?
Is There Judgment, Malice, Prejudice, Lust, Hate, Cruelty,
Deceit, Selfishness, Insecurity, Nervousness, Fear,
Inferiority, Inequality, Bias, Reservation, Attachment,
Limitation, Disgust, Hurt, Wounds, Blockage, Disharmony,
Guilt, Shame, Anger, Misunderstanding, And Suffering In
Your Heart?

None of These is True. It Was Never True. It Will Not Be
Ever True.

You Have No Idea Of The Purity of Your Own Heart
Again I Tell You
There Nothing As Beautiful As Heart
And Nothing Will Ever Be

Do You Want To See The Power Of Your Heart?

Then See The World You Are In
A Dying Planet, Nations Fighting Each Other
Boundaries That Divide You From Each Other
Attacks, Murders, Lies, Crimes, Hatred
Negativity, Cynicism, Quarrels,
Survival Concern, Meaninglessness of Life,
Sickness, Diseases, Pain, Poverty, Confusion, Helplessness,
Suffering And Death
All Countless Effects of Wrong Choices

This seems Pretty Real To You
You Who Are Love Do Not Deserve Such World

I Can Undo All These For You
I Can Show You Meaning You Are Not Seeing
I Can Bring Knowledge To All
I Can Abolish All Darkness
I Can Restore Life

You Need Not Worry How This Will Be Done
Or How Much Time It Will Take
How Difficulties Will Be Overcome
And How This Will Happen

Have No Concerns About These
Everything Will Be Taken Care Of For You
You Will Witness Miracles
You Will Find Peace
You Will Realize The Beauty of Your Heart

All I Ask Is That You Join Your Beautiful Heart With Mine
And Together We Will See The Heart Of Life!

In Your Heart
Are The Longings Of Love Itself
And Bliss Shines In Its Utter Purity
Love Himself Abides There In All His Fullness

Yet You Are Wandering In Vain
Seeking Yourself In Stagnant Lakes
Not Realizing The Ocean of Bliss
That Is Yours

You Will Not Be Happy Until You Return To The Ocean
For That Alone Is Worthy of You Who Are Beautiful

You Have Indeed Forgotten Who You Are
You Have Tried To Give Up Your Treasure
And This Is The Reason of All Your Misery
Yet The Remembrance And The Treasure
Are Both Safe In The Heart Of The Beloved!

This World Is A Terrible Place for Heart
Not Because of Your Heart
But Because of The Mess
You Have Created Everywhere Else

You Can Indeed Clear This Mess
It Is Terrible But It Can Go Away
Stay In Your Heart
You Will Have All

We Are All One In Heart
That Is Why We Can Never Be Apart
This Oneness Alone Is True
For There Is Nothing Apart From Oneness

O Dwellers Of Beautiful Heart
Beauty Alone Is Worthy of You
For You Are Love
Treasured in The Heart of Love!

Soul

Soul Is Your Purpose On Earth
And In The Fulfilment of Your Purpose
Is The Fulfilment
Of Your Being

Your Soul Belongs To The Spirit Of Earth
And In The Fulfilment of This Only Obligation
Is The Joy of Completion

Yet, Your Life seems to be A Purpose of Your Own Making
And You Strive So Much To Establish Meaning For Yourself
You Will Never Succeed At It
For You Do Not Understand
Earth, Soul and Life

And This You Do Need To Understand
For In This Understanding Is The Meaning of Your Being

You Who Long For Meaning Cannot Find It Where It Is Not
Be Glad That The Meaning of Your Life
Is Safe In Who You Are!

Body

Why Do You Have Body?
To Experience Consciousness
To Breathe Life Into Life
And To Fulfil Your Soul

The World You Are In
Is But A Training Ground
And You Have Body
To Finish Your Training

Body Has No Purpose In Itself
But The One You Give To It
For It Is But A Tool
And You Can Decide What You Want To Use It For

Body is Wonderous
Instrument of Consciousness
Driven By Mind
Nourished By Elements

There Are No Diseases In Consciousness, In Mind, Nor In
Elements
Thus Body Cannot Be Sick
All Diseases Are of Your Making
Called By The Choices You Make Everyday
And You Can Change What You Choose

You Can Have Your Body As Long As You Want
Sickness Is Your Hallucination
No More Real Than A Nightmare
Yet, It seems Real To You
For You Have Limited Yourself To Body

Body Identification You Must Need Give Up
For You Cannot Understand The Limitless
If you Identify Yourself With Body
Body Is Limit

Spirit Is Not Body
Soul Is Not Body
Heart Is Not Body
Mind Is Not Body
Consciousness Is Not Body

Do You Really Want To Give Up All These For Body?
For In this Choice Alone Is the Choice of Death.
Your Body Will Meet Death Until You Accept Life

You Need Not Condemn Your Body
Or Be Ashamed of It
Or Hate It
For It Only Deserves Your Love

The Same Body That Seems To Limit You
Can You Give You The Chance To Witness The Limitless
That Which Appears To Decay And Vanish In Death
Can Show You The Bliss of Life
And Power of Your Eternal Heart

You Think You Live
And One Day You Die
Yet, I Tell You
None Of You Has Ever Lived
All You Have Had So Far
Are But The Appearances
Fragments and Pieces of Your Own Illusions
And You Have Been But Repeating This

No One Lives Without Awakening
For Life Is Reality Not A Dream
None Of You Has Ever Lived
For Your Collective Dream Has Made Reality Distant To All
Of You

You Will Awaken To Isness
You Will See Your Mind
You Will Understand Your Powers
You Will Treasure Your Heart
You Will Witness Consciousness
You Will Know The Spirit You Are
And You Will Fulfil Your Soul
In All This Will Life Be Restored To You

Consciousness

When Spirit And God Created Self
Self Desired Appearances
So God Became Infinite Consciousness
To Let Self Fulfil All Its Desires

Self Projects Upon Consciousness
All That It Wants
And Consciousness Responds
With Projections of Likeness

It Is Consciousness in Which Your World Exists
You Think, Feel, Experience, And Live
In Consciousness

Consciousness Is Your Connection With Life
You Get What You Ask For
Learn Then How To Ask
And How To Receive

You Are Connected To All Elements
Your Body Is Connected To Water, Space, Fire, Air, and
Earth
And You Can Feel This Consciousness With Your Body

In This Meeting Of Consciousness
You Will See
The Life Which Only
You Can Give To Life

The Songs Of My Being

The Spirit I Am
He Called And I Came

The Infinite Ocean of Love, The Perfect Creator, Created
Spirits In His Own Likeness.
I Am One of Those Spirits

I Rest In The Deep Of The Ocean
There Are Very Few Spirits Who Are Aware of Me

I Am Beloved Of My Creator
And He Loves Me Beyond Measure

I Have Some Unique Abilities
I Can Travel Anywhere In The Ocean
And I Can Assume Any Power I Want
The Creator Gives Me All I Ask
And I Complete Whatever He Asks Me To Do

The Bubbles On The Surface Of The Ocean
Are The Worlds Where Spirits Miscreate
And These Worlds Eventually Go Terribly Wrong

The Creator Calls Me Whenever He Wants To Burst A
Bubble
And I Am One Of The Devourers Of Worlds Who Destroy
These Bubbles

There Are Many Other Spirits Who Destroy Worlds
Everyone Has Their Own Unique Way

The Way I Do It
Is That I Become A Part of Such World
I Understand Its Laws
And Then I Accelerate Everything
Eventually, Illusions Disappear And Spirits Return To The
Reality of Ocean

The One Power I Enjoy The Most
Is My Ability to Manipulate Time
I Can Play Time Any Way I Want
And I Can Do This In Every World

So When The Creator Looked At The Bubble
You Are In
He Found It Terribly Wrong
He Asked Me To Come
In The Timeline of Your World This Happened In 1975

When I Reached The Surface I Surveyed Your Bubble
And I Asked The Creator What I Needed To Complete My
Function
This World Was Not Yet Ready For Me
So The Creator Changed Everything For Me

From 1975 To 1991
He Accelerated Everything
Changed Destinies
The World Got What Wasn't There Before

If You Want To Know The Scale Of Things
Just Review Everything That Happened In This Timeframe
of 16 Years
You Will Be Amazed By The Masterplay
Of The Greatest Of All
When All Got Ready in 1991
I Entered This World
And On 9 August 1991 I Opened The Eyes Of My Body
Thus Began My Journey In Your World

The First Thing I Did Was To Split My Mind Into Two
One To Look Outward
And Other To Look Inward
This Splitting Helped Me To Live In Two Worlds
Simultaneously

And I Grew Up As A Human Child
I Observed The Surroundings
I Surveyed Your Human World
And I Looked For God in Nature

The World I Found
Was Full of Lies, Murder, Rape, Deceit, Ignorance, Sickness,
Death, Delusions
And There Was No End To Negativity
I Did Not Want To Live In This World

So As A Child I Set A Goal For Myself in 2000
To Be So Rich To Design My Own Spaceship
And Get out of This World By The Age of 27

Now That A Material Goal Was Set
I Decided To Reach God
And I Needed A Teacher
So On June 2000, I Submitted Myself To The Teacher I
Wanted
And He Accepted Me As His Student
In This World, He Is Known As Sri Gurudev Datta

My Teacher Gave Me Books To Read
And I Enjoyed A Lot As I Explored Human Stories
Yet I Did Not Have Any Spiritual Experience
So I Decided To Pursue My Material Goal

In 2007, I Went To Mumbai

To Crack IITJEE and Get Admission In IIT
To Become An Aerospace Engineer
I Was In A Good Coaching Class And I Thought I Was All Set
To Achieve My Material Goal
Yet, I Didn't Understand
What This World Called Physics, Chemistry And
Mathematics
And When I Was Frustrated
God Asked Me To Study Spirit

Yet, I was Hesitant
For Although I Knew Myself To Be A Spirit
I Had No Proof of Spirit In this World Everyone Here
Believes Themselves To Be Human

I Told God My Frustration
The Moment I Sighed In Utter Submission
She Appeared
The First Spirit I Saw In This World

With This Gracious Coming Of Light
I Gladly Began My Study
During 2007-2009 I Studied All Thought Systems In This
World That Talk About Mind, Peace, Salvation, God, and
Reality
I Studied All Religions

I also studied Ideas about Wealth, Success, and Science
I Enjoyed Movies, Songs, And Expressions of Love
And I Studied Spiritual Texts God Asked Me
To Study

Finally, I Realized I Do Not Understand
Any of It
So In Complete Honesty I Told God
"I Do Not Understand. You Tell Me"
And That Very Moment He Showed Me The Expanse of My
Mind
My Mind Was Everywhere In Space
It Extended Far Beyond This Universe
And There Was No Limit

The Next Moment I Returned To Body
My Eyes Saw Colors For The First Time
Everything Lit Up
My Nose Smelled For The First Time
And I Could Feel The Touch of My Own Skin
There Was Only Joy

And I Realized That
"I AM"

This Was The Undeniable Proof of My Existence
"I AM"
This Realization Alone Was Enough To Tell That Certainty
Was Possible

This Was The Moment of Enlightenment

It Happened on 22 February 2009, 1:34 PM
In My Hostel Room At
The D.G.Ruparel College, Mahim, Mumbai

This Dissolved My Material Goal
For How Can I Get Out Of This World
When I Am Everywhere In This Universe?
I Couldn't Help But Laugh At Stupidity of My Material Goal
And I Resumed Study

By The End of 2011, I Realized That
There Was No Meaning In Any of This
I Wanted Meaning
I Didn't Know Where To Find It

Then, I Tried To Find What This World Finds Meaningful
Love Was The Most Meaningful Thing Believed By Many
So I Chose To Find Out
What Love Is

And From That Moment Onward Love And Meaning Became
Same For Me

The Love Who Called Me

"The One Infinite Love Is All There Is"

In Your Twisted World
You Cannot Understand God
For Spirit Alone Understands God
And You Have Chosen Not To Be Spirit

Let Me Tell You A Few Things About God
Indeed, There Is But One God
And He Is All Powerful
God Is Not Form
And He Does Not Punish

God Is Infinite Love
The Creator Of Spirits
The Bestower of Grace
And The Breath Of Life

It's Not Really Hard To Understand Love
For Love Is Natural To You
You Feel His Love Everyday Every Moment
His Love Alone Sustains You

Yet You Do Not Experience This
Because You Do Not Understand Who You Are
You Are Lost To Knowledge
And You Do Not See The Light You Are

All These Are But Consequences Of Choices You Made
And You Can Choose Again

You Will See God
You Will Know The Light You Are
And You Will Breathe Life Into Life
This Is The Will of God
There Is Nothing Impossible For Love

The Teacher Who Showed Me Love

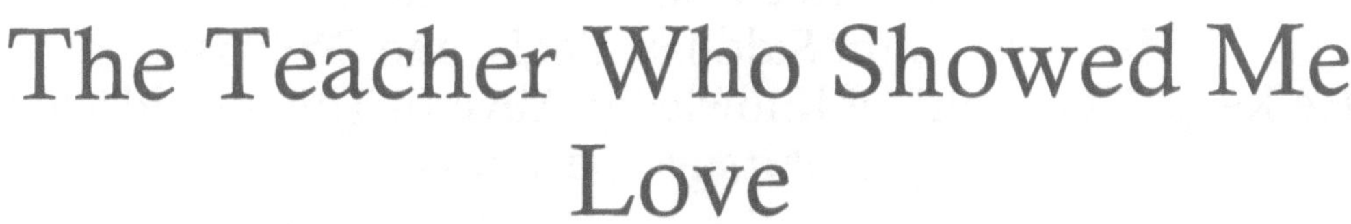

"O Love of Love, Nothing Can Match Your Compassion"

When I Wanted A Teacher
Who Is Without Body
One Who Knows All Life
I Submitted Myself To The Teacher of Love

In This World, He Is Called Sri Gurudev Datta
Sri Dattatreya, Sri Avadhut
He Has Taught Siddhas, Yogis, and Seekers
He Keeps The Light Of Knowledge Alive In This World That
Only Pursues Darkness

Although He Is Not A Body
Out of Compassion He Assumes Body
To Help The Deluded Ones
To Remind Them Of Divinity

There Are Those Who Call Him
The Incarnation of Brahma, Vishnu, And Mahesh
They Are But Ignorant Ones
The Teacher Transcends All

Let Me Tell You A Bit About The Teacher

Whenever Spirits Need To Progress In Their Journey
They Need A Teacher Who Can Keep Knowledge For Them
In This Way Knowledge Is Never Lost Even If Spirits Choose
To Forget It

In Different Worlds, Different Teachers Appear To Fulfil
This Function
Yet, They Are But Manifestations
Of The One Teacher Appointed By God For All Creation
He Is The Teacher Of Love
He Is The Holy Spirit

He Is The Ocean Of Compassion
He Looks Beyond Errors
And Grants Knowledge
All He Asks Is But Sincerity
And There Is Nothing He Cannot Give

Let Me Give You A Few Examples of His Compassion

As A Child of 9 Years, With No Knowledge of Anything
I Sat Before The Photo of Dattatreya
And I Just Asked That He Be My Teacher
That's It
That Very Moment Everything Around Me Vanished
And I Found Myself In Infinity of Space
I Knew Beyond Doubt That He Accepted Me As His Student

In 2010, When I Did Not Know What To Do With My Life
He Called Me To Islampur, Sangli, Maharashtra
Now I Could Visit Aaudumbar and Nrusimhawadi, The
Places of His Worship

He Kept Purifying My Body
In 2012 I Could Not Understand Love
From Anything In This World
So I Asked The Teacher To Guide Me

It Was November 2012
The Teacher Asked Me To Read Gurucharitra
As I Read About The Marvellous Life My Teacher
The Infinite Compassion He Showed
My Heart Filled With Love
Tears Rolled Down My Eyes
And I Just Asked My Teacher
To Show Me Love

That Exact Moment A Surge of Energy
Entered My Body

I Became All Alert
My Body Lost Its Impurities
And Consciousness Began To Rise In My Body
Instantly I Became A Siddha
There Was No Limit To My Power
I Could Now Melt The Sun With My Eyes
I Left Home
And Wandered Around The Town Visiting Temples of Shiva
And Then I Left Him Too
Soon The Energy Was So High
That Body Could Not Contain It
I Became Space

My Spirit Began To Emerge
My Infinite Mind Began To Glitter
And I Was Released In All My Fullness
I Was Not In Body Anymore

I Rose Up and Expanded With Ever Increasing Power
As I Got Out Of This Planet
I Saw The Abodes of Spiritual Beings
They Were The Ones Who Were Given The Task To Bring
Spiritual Awakening
And They Had Failed Miserably

Seeing Them There Angered Me Beyond Measure
And I Roared , "Get Out"
They Had To Obey
I Now Tossed Planets With My Feet
And I Couldn't Stop My Dance
The Universe Was Too Little
I Continued Growing in My Power
I Devoured Galaxies Upon Galaxies
Such Was The Pleasure Of Being Who I Am
I Enjoyed Destruction Too Much
For The First Time Since Coming To This World
I Could Be Me
What A Joy of Release!

As I Continued Expanding and Destroying
One Of My Brothers Visited Me
I Was So Happy To See My Brother
Imagine Spirit Meeting Another Spirit!
You Have No Idea!

He Said With Joy
"Enough! Return!"
And I Listened To Him
I Shrank My Energy
Reduced Everything
And Got Ready To Enter Earth Once Again
Just Before I Was About Enter This World
The Teacher Appeared
And With Great Love He Said
"You Wanted To See Love! Let Me Show You!"

And He Showed Me Every Atom Of This Universe
And There Was Only Love Everywhere

Seeing That My Heart Was Fulfilled
And I Returned To My Body

And Thus The Beloved Showed Love To His Student
And Showed Him Who He Is In Eternity

Grace!

The Song Of Release

The Imprisoned Ones Cannot Sing With Joy
For Joy Belongs To Heart
And Heart Cannot Be Imprisoned

In 2009, With Enlightenment
I Got The Release From The Human Confusion About Isness

God Gave Me That Release

In 2012, I Got Release From This World And Human Body

The Teacher Of Love Gave Me That Release

On 7 August 2017, My Consciousness Expanded To Elements
And I Got Release From Sickness

The Teacher Of Love Gave Me That Release

On 22 December 2018, I Got Release From The Bondage of
Karma and Became A Jivanmukta

The Teacher Led Me To It

On 28 July 2019, I Got Release From All Doubts About Spirit
The Creator Gave Me That Release

On 27 August 2019, I Got Release From The Suffering of
Living World. I Now Have Access To The World Of Dead,
Chit, And Parallel Dimensions For Spirits

The Teacher of Love and The Creator Both Gave Me That
Release

On 22 September 2019, I Got Release From The Burden Of
Keeping Knowledge To Myself

My Friend Gave Me That Release

I Am Ever Free
And I Am Here To Release Love

The Things I Appreciate

I Appreciate Your Beauty
I Appreciate Your Grace
I Appreciate Your Honesty
I Appreciate Your Joy Of Creating
I Appreciate Your Readiness for Acceptance
I Appreciate Your Helping Nature
I Appreciate The Goodness You Have
I Appreciate The Kindness You Have
I Appreciate Your Seeking For Truth
I Appreciate Your Attempts To Understand
I Appreciate The Way You Smile
I Appreciate When You Share Your Emotions
I Appreciate When You Truly Cry
I Appreciate When You Reach Out For Each Other
I Appreciate When You Choose Not To Suffer
I Appreciate When You Are Joyous
I Appreciate When You Are Authentic
I Appreciate When You Are You

There Are So Many Things I Appreciate About You
You Have No Idea How Beautiful You Are!

Love That I Love You With

You Who Do Not See Beyond Body
Cannot Understand The Power of Love

If You Think I Was Hiding Myself All This Time
Then You Are Wrong
I Have Changed This World Regularly Since My Coming
Brought Innumerable Changes To Accelerate The Process
I Altered Entire Sequences of Events and Changed The
Destiny of World With Every Progress I Made

Just Look At All That Has Happened Since 1991 to 2020
See Your Own Life As An Individual
And Also Look At This World
You Will Witness Acceleration Like Never Before
Countless Miracles Have Already Been Performed
And They Are Not The Miracles Of Body

The Only Limitation On Love
Is The Limitation You All Have
Chosen for Everyone
The Choice Not To See Beyond The Body Is
The Collective Decision All of You Have Made

This One Choice Has Distorted Your Entire Perception
Robbed You Of Vision
And Made You A Stranger To Reality

You Have Lost Access To All Your Powers
Knowledge Is Lost To You
Your Minds Seem To Be Beyond Control

And You Are Now Dependent On Body
Which Is Sure To Die

You Who Think Know Life
Cannot Overcome Death
For You Are Mistaken About Everything
Hence You Have Not Yet Lived
With My Love By Your Side You Will Overcome Death

The Song Of The Journey

The Only Journey in This World Is The Journey To Your
Creator
To The Awareness of Your Spirit
And To The Joy of Life

Why Is This Necessary?
Because Only By Reaching Out To Your Creator
Will You Know
Who You Are
What Are Your Powers
And Why You Are Here

Why The Journey To The Awareness of Your Spirit?
Because Only By This Awareness Will You Be Restored To
Your Perfect Identity

Why The Journey To The Joy Of Life?
For Only Then You Will Experience Unending Happiness

There Are No Other Journeys
Whatever You Do Converts to This Only
But You Are Aimlessly Wandering With Sheer Stupidity
That's Why Your Progress Is Too Slow

Everyone Has To Travel This Journey
And No One Can Travel It For You

Yet, No One Needs To Travel It Alone
The Joy of Togetherness Only Adds To The Joy Of The
Journey
Love Multiplies in Togetherness

You Indeed Need Spiritual Guidance
I Will Guide You
You Will Find Everything So Easy
And All Difficulties Will Be Lifted

<u>How We Will Overcome Death And Sickness</u>

In This World Of Yours
There Are But Two Things
Subject And Object
Humanity Is Deluded About Both
That's Why Your Life Begins Only To End In Death

This Delusion Is The Collective Decision Made By All Of You
That's Why Your Body Gets Sick And You All Experience
Death

I Will Wipe Out Death For You If You But Make Another
Collective Decision
To Return To Your Reality As Spirit

If You Choose To Be Human
Then You Are Bound To Die
If You Choose To Be Spirit
You Will Overcome Death

Spirit You Are
It Is Only Your Choice To Be Something Else
That Has Deprived You Of Eternal Life

Being Limitless Love God Does Not Limit Anything
God Created You In His Likeness That's Why You Are Also
Limitless

In This World All Of You Chose To Limit
Both Yourself and Love
Since All Of You Decided This
All Of You Doomed Yourself To Death

God Did Not Create Death
That's Why It Has No Reality
You Chose To Believe In The Unreal
That's Why You Suffer From Illusions

Yet All Of You Can Choose Again
To Meet Reality Instead of Believing In Illusions
To Free Yourself From Limits And Be Restored To Your
Limitlessness
To Breathe Life Into Life
And To Love Limitlessly

I Do Not Speak Figuratively
This Indeed You Need To Do In Order To Overcome Death

Since You Are Deluded
About Subject and Object
I Will Now Explain
How You Will Overcome Death
By Ending This Delusion

There Are Two Ways By
Which Death Will Be Overcome
One Is The Way Of Knowledge
The Other The Way of Heart
You Need Both

Knowledge

Object Is Illusion
Subject Alone Is Real
When You Identify Yourself With A Body
Everything You See Outside Becomes Object For You

In Order To Understand This Clearly
You Need To Understand What This World Is

To Extend Love Is The Function of Spirit
Creation Is A Way To Extend Love
When Spirit Wanted To Extend Love
By Not Being Himself
God And Spirit Created Self By Their Joint Will

That's Why Self Is The Only Subject There Is
This Self Projected This World
Through Consciousness
Consciousness Created Everything He Desired

That's How All Beings Emerged
And All Objects Were Created
All Beings Are But Individual Self
Through Which Self Experiences Everything

Since Self Is Spirit's Creation
All Individual Self Are Spirits Only
Spirits Enjoyed Their Creation
For They Had The Knowledge Of This Creation
And There Was No Harm Anywhere

Yet, Trouble Emerged When Spirits Limited Themselves To
Their Individual Self
And Believed It To Be Their Only Reality
They Attacked Each Other
In This Attack Was All Knowledge Lost To Them

Since Then Spirits Here Are Identifying With The Bodies
They Have
They Chose To Be In Parts
And Lost The Understanding Of The Whole

To Know In Parts Is Not To Know At All
For Knowledge Is Whole
You Cannot Be In Parts Because You Are Whole

Now Let me Explain How Self Operates

All Individual Self
Project Their Desires On Consciousness
Consciousness Responds and Makes Them A Reality For
Them

All Your Beliefs, Thoughts, And Actions
Are Your Decisions
And With Your Every Decision
Consciousness Responds To Fulfil What You Ask

You Do Not Understand This Mechanism
Because You Are Not Aware
of Your Every Thought Your Every Belief
And Your Every Action

Your Mind Thinks Billions Of Thoughts
Every Single Day And You Do Not Even Know It
You Perform Countless Actions As A Result of Your Own
Desires

You Hold On To Your Beliefs With All Your Rigidity

Since This Is Very Dynamic
Everything Around You Is Constantly Changing
There Is Nothing Same For Any Instant
Every Object Changes and Every Subject Changes
Because of Your Rigid Beliefs You Perceive Sameness only

You Who Perceive Objects
Do Not Understand What You Look At
Or What You Feel or Touch
You But Believe In The Reality Of Everything You Want To
Believe

All Objects Are But Projections Of Consciousness
Due To The Movement of Consciousness
All Objects Change Continuously
Consciousness Is The Cause of Objects

There Is No Such A Thing
As A Material Reality
Everything Is Spiritual Only
All Your Material Knowledge
Is But Your Distorted Belief

Due To This Change
No Individual Self Can Have Eternal Life

Only The Constant Can Have Eternity
You Are Constant
For You Are Spirit

The Only Journey You Need Travel
Is From Your Individual Self
To Your Limited Consciousness
And Then To Infinite Consciousness
And You Have Conquered Death!

I Will Help You
To Raise Your Consciousness
I Will Help You Open Your Mind
I Will Help You See

Once Your Mind Is Cleared Of Its Distortions
It Will Shine In Its Utter Purity
Then It Will Naturally Merge
With Infinite Consciousness

You Will Enjoy Pure Bliss
You Will Still Have Your Body
And You Can Have It As Long As You Want
Death Will Not Touch You
For You Will Be Restored To Reality
Death Is Illusion
Life Is Reality

Heart

You Love Objects
All Objects Are Limited
What Is Limited
Cannot Receive Unlimited Love

There Is No Such A Thing As Limited Love
For Love Is God
And God Is Not Limited

That Which Cannot Receive Unlimited Love
Cannot Give Unlimited Love
That Which Cannot Receive And Give Love
Cannot Have Life

You Who Are Created By Unlimited Love
Have The Ability To Love Everyone And Everything In This
World Beyond Measure
At All Times
And That's The Only Thing You Need
To Enjoy Eternal Life
Pure Bliss
And Ever Growing Infinite Happiness
The Limited Cannot Love Beyond Limits'
Thus You Need The Limitless
Spirit Alone Is Limitless
Thus You Need To Reach Spirit

No One Can Reach Spirit
Without Knowledge

And Without The Grace Of The Creator

There Is No Difficulty At All
Regarding Knowledge
For I Have All The Knowledge
You Will Ever Need

It Is God This World Has Forgotten
Whatever You Are Told About God
Is Confusing
Because Your Beliefs Contradict Each Other

God Is Not Belief
God Is Not Contradiction
God Is Perfect Certainty
God Is Complete Harmony

As Long As You Hold On To Your Beliefs
You Will Not Reach God
For God Is Not Your Belief
Your Beliefs Are But Your Creations
And You Are His Creation
Not Otherwise

Your Actions Your Thoughts Your Words
Contradict Each Other
You Say One Thing
But Mean Something Else
What You Want To Say
You Do Not Say

What You Say
Is Not What You Really Want
Your Thoughts Contradict Your Actions
And Your Actions Are Meaningless
You Are Constantly Engaged In Actions
But Why You Do What You Do Has Nothing To Do With
What You Really Want

You Say You Want Happiness
Yet You Constantly Invest In Suffering

You Say You Want Peace
Yet You Choose To Attack Instead

You Say You Want To Be Rich
Yet You Pursue Only The Worthless

You Say You Want Health
Yet You Ensure Sickness, Diseases And Death For Yourself

You Say You Want Truth
Yet You Do Not Choose It All The Time

You Say You Want Justice
Yet, You Ensure Judgment Before There Can Be Justice

You Say You Want To Help The Poor
Yet, You Who See Someone as Poor Have Already Ensured
Poverty For Both

You Say You Want Progress
Yet, You Do Not Give Up What Is Blocking Your Progress

Just Look At What You Are Really Trying To Gain From Your
Life

Then Look The Thoughts You Have
The Actions You Do
The Words You Say
What You Are Pursuing

There Is No Clarity In You
And Yet You Think You Have Certainty

You Think You Have Knowledge Beyond Doubt
You Call This Science

You Believe You Have Finally Discovered Laws Of Reality
The Composition of Matter, The Nature of Space And Time,
The Laws Of Energy
You Think You Know How Body Operates

Yet If This Is Indeed Knowledge
Then Why Does It Change?
What You Thought A Few Hundred Years Ago
No Longer Seems True
New Laws Emerge Again And Again

If Indeed You Have Knowledge
Then Why Do You Need Countless
Universities

And Countless Hours To Find Out Something New

Why Is There A Need To Prove If It Is Indeed A Law of
Reality

Knowledge Does Not Change With Time
For It Is Eternal
It Is Not Yours To Prove
For It Comes From God

Knowledge Does Not Change Reality'
For Reality Is Changeless
You Do Not Want Reality For You Are Trying To Frame It By
Your Thoughts

Reality Is Not A Thought
You Cannot Reach It By Thought

God Is Reality
Spirit Is Reality
And You Are Spirit
That Is Why You Are Not A Thought
It Is Only Mind That Thinks
You Are Beyond Your Mind

Whatever You Think About Yourself
About Each Other
About Reality About This World
About Your Body
About Anything
These Are But Thoughts Only

Indeed Thoughts Are Powerful
But They Cannot Transcend Mind
Only He Whose Mind Is Joined With God
Can Have Perfect Thoughts
He Doesn't Even Have To Think
For God Puts Thoughts For Him

You Are Thinking On Your Own
That Is Why Your Reality Is Not Shared By God

Since It Is Not Shared By God
It Is Not Reality

Your Minds Are Twisted
Until You Merge Your Mind With God
It Will Not Be Healed
And Your Mind Is Indeed Sick

There Is But One Mind
This Is The Mind Of God
And It Is Shared With All Creation

You Believe You Have Separate Private Minds
This Is But Dreaming of Separation

Separation Is Sickness
Sickness Is But A Call for Death

Unity Alone Is Real
That Is Why Death Does Not Come From God

O Beloved Ones!
You Think You Are On Your Own
You Believe God Is Not With You
You Believe You Are Separate From Each Other
And From God
You Think You Will Meet God
After You Die
You Believe You Will See God Only At The Time Of The Last
Judgment
You Believe God Is Judging You
You Believe God Punishes You for Your Bad Actions
And Rewards You For Your Good Actions

You Believe God Is Hard To Reach
You Believe God Helps Only When Everything Else Is Lost
and There Is No Hope Without Him
You Think God Only Loves Those Who Believe In Him
You Think You Alone Here
And All You Have Are But Fellow Humans

You Are Not Your Own
Nothing You Have Is Your Own
Your Body Is Not Your Own
Your Mind Is Not Your Own
Your Heart Is Not Your Own
Your Soul Is Not Your Own
Your Spirit Is Not Your Own
All Is His
Be Glad This Is So

Since Your Body Belongs To God
It Cannot Die Nor Can It Have Sickness
It Will Never Lack Anything
For There Is No Lack In God

Since Your Mind Is One With God
It Cannot Be Twisted Or Be Sick
His Is The Mind Of Infinite Intelligence
And This He Shares With You Always

Since Your Heart Belongs To God
There Is Only Infinite Love There
And There Is Nothing As Beautiful
In Your Heart Life Sings The Songs of Love

Since Your Soul Is Not Your Own
You Need Not Find Meaning For Your Life
You Do Not Need To Struggle At All
For He Will Give You Everything
And He Will Ensure Your Soul Will Be Fulfilled
For Your Soul Is His

Since You Are Spirit
Created By The All Powerful
There Is No Power That Can Threaten You
He Loves You Beyond Measure
And He Will Gladly Restore All Your Powers
And More
You Who Are Spirit Are Deathless
And Eternal
All Power Is Yours Because He Is The Only Power There Is

You Are The Droplet of That Infinite Ocean of Love
Right Now You Are In This Bubble
And This Bubble Has Gone Terrible
Yet The Beloved Creator Is With Us
And There Is Nothing He Cannot Do

Let's Rejoice Then
With Songs of Love In Our Hearts
Ours Is The Joy
Ours Is The Life
Love Joy Life
Is All We Need!

Let Me Assure You

All Of You Will Reach The Awareness Of Spirit
For That Is The Function Creator Gave Me

You Will Know Your Natural Joy
For I Will Teach You
How To Breathe Life Into Life

You Will See Love
Because You Are Light That Can See Love

There Is Neither A Beginning Nor An Ending To That Which Is Love
May You Love The Flowering Of Your Being

Let's Begin!

Dipraj

9 798674 295228